The HCG Guidebook

Your Key to Weight Loss &
Other Hidden Benefits

Felicia Weiss, Ph.D.
&
Tony Cecala, Ph.D.

The HCG Guidebook

Dedication

This book is dedicated to our children, Marissa and Joel.

Acknowledgements

We would like to thank Cynthia Novak for introducing us to HCG and for all of her support and guidance over the years. We also wish to acknowledge Irene Weiss for her love, support and enthusiasm for this program. Thank you, Dr. Angel Russo, for reading the manuscript and providing excellent feedback. You are a gifted psychologist and an incredible friend.

Finally, we would like to thank our customers, who amaze us daily with their results and accomplishments and who inspired us to write this book.

Table of Contents

Chapter 10
Sharing HCG Diet Experiences 87

Foreword

It is our goal in writing this book to share the work of Dr. A.T.W. Simeons in his manuscript "Pounds and Inches" and to help make the HCG program easy to understand and follow. Having done this program successfully ourselves and having worked with several hundred people, who have also achieved their weight loss goals, we have gathered a "bookload" of valuable information on how to do the HCG program correctly. Although there are many diets available, we have found this one to be the most effective, convenient, affordable and gratifying program we have ever seen. We wish to share this knowledge with those who are considering this program or who have already made a decision to do it.

Felicia is trained and licensed as a clinical psychologist. Tony is a cognitive psychologist, who specializes in user interface design. We have long had an interest in the natural health field. In 1992 we began publishing our free guide to wellness and personal growth in the Dallas/Fort Worth area called the "Holistic Networker". In 1994 we began producing the Wellness Expo®. We also produce a website at: www.HolisticNetworker.com which contains many valuable articles and a directory of holistic practitioners from around the world. The website for our products company, Shifting Frequencies, is at www.ShiftingFrequencies.com where the homeopathic HCG drops we are discussing in this book are available. We have been fortunate in learning about many groundbreaking technologies over the years and enjoy sharing them with others.

Preface

Who is this book for?

If what you have been doing was working for you, then you would not be reading this. This book is for people who are ready and willing to make a positive change in their lives and to take back control of their bodies. Your body is your vehicle. If you take good care of it and treat it well, then it can take you on your journey in the best possible way. If you have tried many other diets and failed or if you weigh more than you would like and feel this could be a quick and comfortable way to achieve your weight loss goals, then this program may be for you. Of course, we recommend checking with your doctor before starting any kind of weight loss program, especially if you have health issues or concerns.

Medical Disclaimer

Whenever considering a weight loss program, consult with your healthcare provider. The information provided here is not intended to replace consultation or advice received by qualified health professionals regarding your specific situation nor is it to be taken as medical advice or diagnosis. All information offered in this book is based on the protocol proposed by Dr. Simeons, as well as our personal experiences and that of several hundred others we have worked with.

HCG: The Controversy and the Results

Since 1975, the FDA has required labeling and advertising of HCG to state: "HCG has not been demonstrated to be an effective adjunctive therapy in the treatment of obesity. There is no substantial evidence that it increases weight loss beyond that resulting from caloric restriction, that it causes a more attractive or 'normal' distribution of fat, or that it decreases the hunger and discomfort associated with calorie-restricted diets." This does not mean it's not safe or effective. It simply means that there are no peer-reviewed, double-blind clinical studies that support the use of HCG as a dietary aid.

Chapter 1

How it All Began
The Remarkable Work of Dr. A.T.W. Simeons

Abstract

Dr. Simeons has contributed a breakthrough in the field of obesity and weight control. Thanks to his discovery of the role of HCG in weight management, we now have a scientific approach to weight loss that works comfortably and consistently for people. He was truly a pioneer, whose work is incredibly beneficial and helpful in solving the obesity problem that has grown to epic proportions in the United States.

Pounds and Inches

Dr. A.T.W. Simeons was a British Endocrinologist, who spent decades studying the nature and treatment of obesity. In the late 1930s after looking at thousands of cases and developing a treatment that showed good results, Dr. Simeons began publishing his findings in scientific journals. However, he received so many inquiries from research institutes, doctors, and patients that in 1954 he published a manuscript called

"Pounds and Inches" to explain his findings to both laypersons and professionals.

Three Types of Fat

First, he discussed the nature of obesity, a disorder he believed can be inherited. Then he distinguished among three types of fat: 1. structural- which provides the important and necessary function of filling the gaps between various organs; 2. normal reserve of fuel- which is utilized for muscular activity and the maintenance of body temperature; and 3. abnormal reserve of fuel—which is locked away and unavailable to the body in a nutritional emergency. While the first two types of fat are necessary for our survival, it is the latter type that can lead to obesity and that is difficult to lose during normal dieting. After studying various glands and brain function, Dr. Simeons concluded that it is the hypothalamus (the part of the brain from which the central nervous system controls all the autonomic functions of the body, such as breathing, heart beat, digestion, etc.), which manages the deposits and withdrawals of fat. When a person consumes more fat than their body requires, the hypothalamus locks it away and takes it out of normal circulation.

Three Paths to Becoming Overweight

This discovery led Dr. Simeons to conclude that there are three basic ways for a person to become overweight or even obese. First, they might have inherited an abnormally low fat-banking capacity. Second, their prior normal fat-banking capacity may have been lowered due to some other disorder of their hypothalamus, such as might occur in menopause or some types of diabetes. Finally, obesity can occur when a normal fat-center is suddenly required to handle more food than is needed for momentary requirements (such as when a person overeats, exercises less, etc.). Dr. Simeons noted that in the first two situations, obesity may occur regardless of whether a person overeats. He reasoned that, to treat obesity, he had to correct any hypothalamic deficiencies.

HCG: The Key to Weight Loss

Dr. Simeons understood that pregnant women have enormous quantities of Human Chorionic Gonadotrophin (HCG) circulating in their bodies. This allows pregnant women to experience almost unlimited hypothalamic banking capacity so that fat deposits are not formed. This is how the fetus is able to gain nourishment even if the mother is not eating. After she gives birth and the HCG is gone, a formerly pregnant women's hypothalamus reverts to its normal capacity so that abnormally accumulated fat is locked away and banked and obesity may once again occur.

Dr. Simeons discovered that by injecting a person with HCG and restricting them to a very low calorie diet (since they don't have a baby growing inside of them) that they could access their fat stores and lose weight. He found that HCG seems to continually saturate the blood, allowing people to not feel hungry, although their food intake has been drastically reduced. Since HCG is not a sex hormone, it operates the same way in men, women and children.

Complicating Disorders

Dr. Simeons' noted that there are many disorders often associated with obesity. The ones where obesity seems to play a precipitating or aggravating role are: the stable type of diabetes, gout, rheumatism and arthritis, high blood pressure and hardening of the arteries, coronary disease and cerebral hemorrhage. He noted that it is very important for people with these conditions to be monitored by a doctor when doing the HCG diet as their condition may improve as they lose weight.

Dr. Simeons' HCG Clinic in Italy

Dr. Simeons successfully applied his new approach to weight loss to thousands of patients in his clinic in

Italy. He recommended that patients take the HCG for 23-40 days. He had the HCG administered to them by injection. After the injections were stopped, he had his patients continue with their low-calorie diet for three more days to be sure that all the HCG was eliminated from their body. He found that his patients were no more hungry during these three days than while taking the HCG.

HCG and "Loading Days"

For the first two days with the HCG, Dr. Simeons had his patients eat large quantities of fatty and sugary foods. He felt these "loading" days were important to swell the fat stores in their body so that when the low-calorie diet was begun that these fat stores would be more easily accessed. With reasonably well-stocked fat reserves, Dr. Simeons' patients were able to comfortably be on a 500 calorie/day diet. Although his patients would often gain a few pounds on their two loading days, they generally lost all of this weight in the first 48 hours of the low-calorie diet. Then they tended to lose ½ to 1 pound/day of fatty tissue for the duration. Since they were losing their fat stores and not their structural fat or normal fat reserves, they found that their weight loss occurred in the areas where they needed to lose it the most.

The Transition Phase of the HCG Diet

Following their program, Dr. Simeons' patients entered a transition phase for the next three weeks. During this transition phase, they could eat whatever they chose, with the exception of sugars and starches. He encouraged them to weigh themselves daily and to make appropriate modifications if they gained more than two pounds. After this transition phase, they were able to slowly add other foods, and, importantly, to continue their daily weighing. Overall, he found that 60-70% of his patients experienced little or no trouble in permanently maintaining their weight loss. He noted that many of his patients who regained weight did so as a result of not continuing to weigh themselves daily and to make adjustments as needed. Dr. Simeons found that patients who had more weight to lose or who had regained some of their weight were able to do additional rounds of the HCG program quite successfully and comfortably. Dr. Simeons just recommended that a person wait at least six weeks before starting a second round. He felt if more courses of the program were necessary, a person should wait for longer intervals each time. He recommended eight weeks between a second and third round, twelve weeks between a third and fourth round, twenty weeks between a fourth and fifth round, and six months between a fifth and sixth course. In this way a person can lose over 100 pounds, if they needed, without experiencing difficulty.

Two Types of HCG

Although Dr. Simeons focused solely on HCG injections, today HCG is also available in homeopathic form. The advantage to this is that the HCG homeopathic drops are more easily administered (the drops are just held under the tongue for about 30 seconds and then swallowed) and they are very inexpensive. Many have found them to be equally effective to the HCG injections. We have found them to work quite well and have known many people, including ourselves, who have used them successfully to achieve their weight loss goals. It is important to make sure that the homeopathic HCG drops are manufactured by a reputable manufacturer, who manufactures them according to the strictest standards in a federally- and state-registered pharmaceutical laboratory, which has regular inspections by the Food and Drug Administration (FDA) in order to ensure compliance with current Good Manufacturing Practices (cGMP) and the Code of Federal Regulations (CFR).

Chapter 2

What is Homeopathy?

The basic principle of homeopathy, known as the "law of similars", is "let like be cured by like." It was first stated by German physician Samuel Hahnemann in 1796. Homeopathy has been widely used throughout the world for more than 200 years. Homeopathy has been available in the UK since the mid-1800s. It began as a medicine for the elite, in fact the British Royal Family employs a homeopathic physician to this day. In fact, we have heard that members of the British Royal Family take their homeopathic first aid kit with them when they travel. In general, it has been found that homeopathy can be safely used with conventional medicines and that it will not interfere with the action of medicines prescribed by your doctor. Since homeopathic medicines (often referred to as remedies) are non-toxic, there are no serious side effects and they are safe.

Based upon a review of 20 studies (including 7,275 patients), the European Council for Classical Homeopathy found no cases of serious adverse events or serious adverse drug reactions (January 2009). The results of randomized clinical trials in observational studies have also confirmed that homeopathic treatment does not result in any serious adverse effects and is safe. This is due to the fact that, unlike conventional medicines, homeopathic medicines are highly-diluted.

Zofia Dymitr, the Society of Homeopaths Chairwoman said: "Homeopathy is an evidence-based medicine and there is plenty of research supporting its efficacy beyond placebo. There is also evidence that homeopathy is cost effective." Zofia added: "While it is true that science cannot yet explain the precise mechanism of action of ultra high dilutions such as homeopathic medicines, this does not mean that there is no mechanism of action." For more information about homeopathy research please visit the Society of Homeopaths website at www.homeopathy-soh.org

The homeopathic HCG drops are made by starting with a small amount of HCG. This HCG solution is diluted until it no longer contains even a single molecule of HCG. The "energy signature" or frequencies of the HCG remains in a solution of alcohol.

We have found these homeopathic HCG drops to be highly effective. Although we have not had the HCG injections ourselves and cannot speak about them from personal experience, we have spoken with several people who have tried both the injections and the

HCG homeopathic drops. The people we have spoken with have told us that they have preferred the homeopathic HCG drops for several reasons. First, they are much less expensive. Second, they are very convenient and do not involve receiving or self-administering a daily injection. Third, since the injection is administered only once/day, some have found that their appetite is not suppressed to the extent it is with the homeopathic drops as these are generally self-administered about three times/day. Finally, one person reported to us that she had gotten an infection from the injections. Of course, the people we have spoken with have said that they did quite well and lost a lot of weight with the HCG injections and so their efficacy is certainly well-established. We also recognize that some people prefer to be under a doctor's daily supervision and, in fact, they may have health issues that warrant this. We have the utmost respect for medical doctors and always encourage people to check with their doctor before starting any weight loss or detox program.

We have had a long history of success with homeopathy and are convinced of its efficacy. Over eighteen years ago, when our daughter was an infant, she was very irritable and would get a fever when she was teething. At that time a friend introduced us to chamomilia, which is a homeopathic remedy that helps with this issue. She gave it to us in liquid form in a bottle with a dropper, which we administered to our daughter. We noticed that her fever rapidly disappeared and her fussiness also went away. Our daughter loved taking her dropper of chamomilia since it tasted like water. In fact, we found that if we attempted to give her some children's Tylenol that she would reject it. This surprised us as it did have a sweet grape taste. We were impressed that she intuitively gravitated to the homeopathic remedy.

A few years later we were introduced to the homeopathic remedy Arnica Montana, which is good for physical injuries, such as sprains, and bumps. When our son was only about two-years-old, he fell and banged his forehead very hard on a table. His forehead began to turn red. We immediately gave him some Arnica Montana in pellet form. We told him to hold these under his tongue until they dissolved. He happily took what he called "the white medicine", which is relatively tasteless and dissolves in your mouth. To our surprise, in about 15 minutes the redness on his forehead had disappeared completely and he never developed a bruise. Since then everyone in our family has used the Arnica Montana with great results. We have since learned that it is also available as a gel and we keep both in our home at all times. Whenever any of us experiences a physical injury, we make sure to use it.

A friend told us recently that her sister had had a hysterectomy. Afterwards, she had taken the medicine her doctors prescribed and, she also took Arnica Montana. Her doctors told her that they had never seen such a rapid recovery.

Finally, we have been amazed at our results and the results of hundreds of others we have known with the HCG homeopathic drops. We are firmly convinced of their effectiveness. Sometimes we have people order just one small bottle of homeopathic HCG so they can give this a try. Invariably they end up ordering more. Often they send their family, friends and co-workers to buy their bottles as now they, too, are ready to do this program. Once they have completed the program, if they have more weight to lose, they come back to do it again.

Having been involved in the holistic health field for almost 20 years, we have learned of so many wonderful alternatives to traditional medicine. Of course, we appreciate the value of traditional medicine and find that often the two are complementary. We always say, if you break your leg, then it is good to see a doctor to have it set and a cast put on. However, you might also wish to have some energy work or some other form of natural healing done on it as well. You will most likely benefit from taking Arnica Montana, too. We believe that it is important to be open to what is out there and to see what feels right and works well for you.

Chapter 3

Details of the HCG Diet

Days 1 and 2: The Loading Days

Dr. Simeons found that it is important for a person to eat to capacity lots of fatty and sugary foods on these first two days. It is essential to take the homeopathic HCG drops or to get the HCG injections on these days as well. This can be an enjoyable experience for people who have been depriving themselves and is an important first phase of the program. It is also a good opportunity to indulge yourself and to allow yourself the chance to consume the foods you may love, but usually do not allow yourself to experience. You can have a lot of fun with this phase. You can plan ahead and buy your favorite foods, go to an all you-can-eat buffet, eat pizza, have ice cream and other rich desserts, etc. Of course, if you have any health issues that would make this unhealthy for you, then check with your doctor and figure out an appropriate way for you to load. You may wish to consume lots of nuts, avocado, pineapple, and other high-fat, high carbohydrate foods that are healthier for you.

Ironically, because the HCG takes away a lot of a person's appetite, these two loading days may not be as easy as they sound. Psychologically, as you feel full to capacity you may realize that consuming these foods is not as enjoyable as you thought it would be. The weight gain you experience and other unpleasant physical sensations such as feeling bloated, tired, etc., may help you to see that eating lots of fatty and sugary foods is not all that you expected it to be. This can help you to feel excited to begin the low calorie part of the program on Day 3 and to get your cravings for many of these foods out of your system.

The 500-calorie Diet

On day 3 you begin the 500-calorie diet, which you will continue for 23 to 40 days. Although 500 calories sounds like very little food, we have actually found it to be quite filling and much more food than you would expect. This is because the HCG helps to eliminate most of your hunger and you feel full quickly. Also, since you are also accessing your fat stores, you really are not just living on 500 calories/day. Many people find that they have lots of energy and feel quite good while in this low-calorie phase, especially if they have done their two loading days correctly.

We have not found it necessary to rigidly count calories each day. If you only eat the allowed foods in the quantities specified then you will naturally stay within the caloric guidelines.

Breakfast

You can have tea or coffee in any quantity without sugar. You can use Stevia or some other artificial sweetener. You can also have one tablespoon of milk in a 24-hour period. (You can also have a piece of fruit and/or a breadstick or piece of melba toast if you deduct it from your lunch or dinner).

Lunch

1. You can have 100 grams (about 3.5 ounces) of veal, beef, chicken breast, fresh white fish, lobster, crab, or shrimp. It is important to remove all the visible fat before cooking and the meat is weighed when it is still raw. You can boil or grill it without adding any additional fat.

2. You can have one type of vegetable only from the following list: spinach, chard, chicory, beet-greens, green salad, tomatoes, celery, fennel, onions, red radishes, cucumbers, asparagus and cabbage. (Since most vegetables have very few calories, you do not have to weigh these items and are not limited to a set amount. It is just good not to go overboard.)

3. One breadstick (grissino) or one Melba toast.

4. An apple or a handful of strawberries or one-half grapefruit. The size of the apple does not matter as long as only one apple is consumed at a time.

Dinner

Here you get to have the same choices as lunch. Of course, it is good to choose a different protein and vegetable.

You are also allowed the juice of one lemon daily, as well as salt, pepper, vinegar, mustard powder, garlic, sweet basil, parsley, thyme, majoram, etc., for seasoning. Just avoid any oil, butter or dressing.

You are able to drink tea, coffee, plain water, and diet soda in any quantity and at all times. It is important to drink about two liters of water per day.

You can break up your two meals however you would like as long as you do not have your two breadsticks or two pieces of fruit at one time. The fruit and breadstick can be eaten between meals or for breakfast instead of with lunch or dinner. It is just important that you not eat more than the four items listed at one meal. Also, any food you did not eat from the previous day cannot be added on the following day.

While on this program, it is best to avoid cosmetics other than lipstick, eyebrow pencil and powder. If you are taking medication, then consult with your doctor. Fortunately, most medicines do not interfere with the HCG homeopathic drops and vice versa. In terms of lotions, you want to avoid all lotions that contain animal or vegetable fats. Unfortunately, most lotions contain these substances. The only kind of lotion you are able to use are ones that are made with mineral oil. This is because animal and vegetable fats are absorbed through your skin and will affect the success of your program. If you are unable to locate a lotion with mineral oil, then it is best to protect yourself from the sun while on the program either with a hat, pants, and/or long sleeves, by staying in the shade as much as possible, or by remaining indoors. Here you can remind yourself that it is just for a few weeks. Personally, we have found that your skin is fairly moist while on the program and does not seem to require the usual amount of lotion so this is not really as much of a hardship as you might think. Of course, we are firm believers in sun screen and so we do consider protecting yourself against the sun to be very important during the program when you are not able to use your usual protection.

Here is a sample menu:

Breakfast Menu

- Coffee with one tablespoon of milk and Stevia.
- One-half grapefruit with Stevia.
- One breadstick (Torinese grissino)

Lunch Menu

- 100 grams (3.5 ounces) of chicken breast
- green salad (lettuce and balsamic vinegar)
- water, coffee, tea, or any diet beverage

Dinner Menu

- 100 grams (3.5 ounces) of steak
- tomatoes
- water, coffee, tea, or any diet beverage

After Dinner Snack

- 1 apple
- 1 breadstick
- 1 cup of herbal tea sweetened with stevia

As you can see, this is actually a fair amount of food. Most people find it quite filling and satisfying. Of course, it is important to take your HCG on these day or this amount of food would not feel like enough. Also, it is good to make sure to stay within the 500 calories and to make your choices accordingly. (Therefore, it is fine to have steak once/day, however, twice/day would be too high in calories.)

Dr. Simeons recommended that menstruating women ideally should begin the HCG program immediately after a period. If this is not possible, then he recommended being on the program at least 10 days before their period is due. During menstruation a woman should stop the HCG, while continuing on the diet. Most women do not feel any more hungry on these days. However, it is best to wait until your period actually comes before stopping the HCG so that you can remain on the 500-calorie diet comfortably. Once your period is over, you would begin taking the HCG again. Dr. Simeons explained that if you are nearing the end of a round of the program and your period is approaching, that it is best to stop the HCG at least three days before you begin menstruating. If you have gotten your period in the middle of doing the program and have had to stop taking the HCG, then it is best to continue it for at least three days after menstruating before stopping.

If you should experience a "plateau" on this program, which Dr. Simeons defined as when you go 4-6 days without losing any weight, this will correct itself. If, however, you feel that you need to do something about this just to feel better psychologically, then Dr. Simeons recommended an "apple day". This would begin at lunch and continue until just before lunch on the next day. Here you would eat up to six large apples when you desire one. Dr. Simeons found that most people did not need to drink any water while doing this, however, he said a person could drink a little water if needed if they did feel thirsty. Other than this, he suggested they not eat or drink anything else. He did state that a person would only do an apple day on a day when they are taking the HCG and only if they had reached a plateau and were unwilling to wait for it to resolve itself naturally. Therefore, if a person is not taking the HCG because they are menstruating or if it is one of their last three days without the HCG, then they would refrain from doing an apple day. Dr. Simeons found that an apple day tends to result in a fair amount of weight being lost the next day, mostly because of the elimination of water, and then the weight loss tends to continue when a person has resumed their normal 500-calorie diet.

Once you have completed the 23-40 days with the HCG, then you will want to stop taking it while continuing on the low calorie diet for three more days. This is to ensure that the HCG is completely out of your system. You should not feel any more hungry on these last three days as you did while taking the HCG because it is still in your body.

The Transition Phase

Now you are ready for the Transition Phase, which lasts for three weeks. It is very similar to the Atkins-type diet. It involves eating anything you please, as long as you avoid sugar and starch, and as long as you continue to weigh yourself daily as soon as you wake up and have emptied your bladder. If you gain more than two pounds, then Dr. Simeons recommended doing a "steak day". This is where you cut back and skip breakfast and lunch, while drinking a lot of fluids. Then for dinner he suggested eating a huge steak with only an apple or raw tomato. In fact, Dr. Simeons felt it was very important that a person do this steak day on the same day that their morning weight registered a weight gain of more than two pounds. He found that the next day a person usually would lose a pound or more and be back on track.

Dr. Simeons found that many people are surprised at how small their appetite has become and yet how much they can eat without gaining weight in this phase. They tend to stop suffering from an abnormal appetite and usually feel satisfied with much less food than before. While it is important not to gain more than two pounds during this phase, it is equally important not to lose more than two pounds. The reason for this is that a greater loss of weight is achieved at the expense of normal fat. He found that this lost fat was invariably regained as soon as more food was eaten resulting in a gain of more than two pounds.

The Maintenance Phase

After your three weeks of transition, you are ready to begin the maintenance phase. Here it is good to start adding back regular foods slowly. Continue weighing yourself each day and observe how you feel after consuming these foods. Which foods cause you to gain weight? How do you feel after eating gluten or sugar? If you gain more than two pounds, then it is a good idea to cut back immediately and/or to avoid the foods that are causing your weight gain. If your weight continues to go higher, then Dr. Simeons recommended that a person do a "steak day" (the same way as in the transition phase), where you would skip breakfast and lunch while having plenty to drink. Then for dinner you would eat a huge steak with only an apple or a raw tomato.

As in the transition phase, Dr. Simeons discovered that not only was it important for people not to gain more than two pounds while in the maintenance phase, it is also better for them not to lose more than two pounds.

Chapter 4

Shopping and Planning

One of the benefits of this program is that it takes away much of your appetite so that you are able to be comfortable eating only 500 calories/day. You will find that you save money on groceries during this low-calorie phase.

The Loading Days

It is important that you eat lots of sugary and fatty foods on the first two days of this program, while taking the HCG. Although you will gain some weight doing this, you are able to lose this weight usually within the first two days of doing the low calorie part of this diet. By doing your loading properly, however, you will expand your fat cells, making it easier for your body to access them and you will be more comfortable when on the low calorie part of this diet.

Think about what your favorite foods are. It is a good idea to go to the store and buy them, to go out to dinner, to get ice cream, bake cookies, have pizza, etc., (as long as you don't have any health reasons not to do this). If for health reasons you are not able to eat like this, then get foods that are high in fat, such as nuts, avocados, pesto and cheeses, but that are somewhat healthier for you. If you wish to avoid sugars, then focus on fats. The important thing is that you get lots of fats and/or sugars during this two day period.

The HCG Low-Calorie Phase

Whether or not a vegetable is canned seems to make no difference when on this program. Of course, it is always better to have fresh vegetables when possible, but many of us lead busy lives and may not have the time to shop for and cook fresh vegetables each day. It is a good idea when shopping that you carefully read labels. Pay attention to sugars and oils that may be contained in an item you might not expect. For example, some brands of salsa or diced tomatos contain sugars and oils, while others do not. You want to avoid these sugars and oils as they will make it difficult for you to do this program successfully.

When purchasing apples, you can buy large ones if you like. According to Dr. Simeons, the size of the apple does not matter. The important thing is that you eat only one apple at a time. Keep in mind that two small apples will not replace one large one. So it is better to buy larger apples if you wish to consume more food.

You will also want to buy your protein and vegetables. Personally, we found it filling to have steak or beef once/day. Do your best to find proteins that are lean as you will have to remove any visible fats.

Shopping carefully during Phase 2 is essential to success. We know, because we ourselves have had days where we assumed we would lose weight, and later realized that our gain was due to hidden sugar in a can of diced tomatoes. Check your labels carefully! Sugar has many names: agave nectar, barley malt, buttered syrup, cane-juice crystals, caramel, carob syrup, corn syrup, corn syrup solids, dextran, dextrose, diatase, diastatic malt, ethyl maltol, fructose, fruit juice, fruit juice concentrate, glucose, glucose solids, golden syrup, HFCS, high-fructose corn syrup, honey, invert sugar, lactose, malt syrup, maltodextrin, maltose, mannitol, molasses, refiner's syrup, sorbitol, sorghum syrup, and sucrose. We recommend a natural non-caloric herbal sweetener called "stevia". The Stevia leaf is naturally super-sweet; only a few drops or crystals of stevia go a long way. Some people find that they don't care for the flavor of stevia. For those people we suggest finding an artificial sweetener. The three primary compounds used as sugar substitutes in the United States are saccharin (e.g., Sweet'N Low), aspartame (e.g., Equal, NutraSweet) and sucralose (e.g., Splenda, Altern). Many in the natural health community will scoff at the mention of these. We, however, look at the global pattern of ongoing obesity and weight-related illnesses and believe these sweeteners to be the "lesser of two evils".

Shopping for meat can also have its challenges. If you look closely on prepared chicken, seafood, and beef labels you will sometimes find that corn syrup and other sweeteners have been added. Remember, when you purchase meat, the label should read 0 (zero) carbohydrates.

Approved whitefish and seafood choices may contain up to 1 gram of fat. Red meats, however, can be very fatty. Think about your lean ground hamburger meat, even a "93/7" lean/fat rated ground beef has about 7 to 9 grams of fat in 3.5 ounces. That's why we recommend eating lean cuts such as trimmed top round, eye round, petite sirloin, or extra lean stew meat. A porterhouse, t-bone, or rib eye steak is going to be a lot of trouble to trim. We recommend saving these cuts for Phase 3 of the program where you can consume the extra fat without too much concern.

The Transition Phase

This phase lasts for three weeks. The reason for this is that Dr. Simeons found that it takes about three weeks before the weight reached at the end of the low-calorie phase becomes stable.

We greatly enjoy the transition phase. Here you can eat whatever you like as long as you avoid sugars and starches. You are now able to add items like nuts, cheeses, and eggs to your diet. At the same time, it is important to avoid fruits that contain a lot of natural sugar and carbohydrates, so apples are no longer recommended at this stage. (By now most people are willing to give apples up for a few weeks as they have consumed so many during the low-calorie part of this program). You can have a ½ cup of strawberries, some blueberries, blackberries, and other fruits once/day as long as they are low in carbohydrates and natural sugars.

Heavy cream has zero carbohydrates. You can use this to make your own whipped cream. All you do is whip it with some stevia or other natural sweetener and you have a delicious whipped cream you can pour over your fruit for a dessert once/day. Land O'Lakes even makes a sugar-free whipped cream that is made with heavy cream and contains zero carbohydrates. It has a purple top and can sometimes be found at Wal-Mart and other grocery stores.

Dr. Simeons found that as long as no carbohydrates are eaten during this phase, then fats can be indulged in more liberally. Even small quantities of alcohol, such as an occasional glass of wine with a meal, are allowed. However, it is important to avoid sugars and starches during this phase because Dr. Simeons found that when starches and fats are combined during these first three weeks that things can get out of hand and weight can be regained.

We have noticed after completing the HCG program that we do not have the sugar cravings we had before. Also, although we choose to sometimes have a little sugar after the transition phase has been completed, we do not indulge ourselves the way we used to. You may find that you, too, feel so good when not eating sugar that it is not something you wish to return to in the same way you did before.

The Maintenance Phase

The Maintenance Phase is perhaps the most importance phase—this is how you decide to eat for the rest of your life. By the time you start this phase, you will know that you can actually go for weeks on end without feeling the need for a "sugar high". To maintain all your wonderful wins on the program, your relationship with sugar, starches, and empty carbohydrates will need to be different.

It all begins at the grocery store. Do you really want to swing by the bakery section? Do you need to eat sugary cereals? Are all those sauces, condiments, and snacks filled with high-fructose corn syrup really needed? Of course, the answer is "no", but how do we find a healthy balance? How do we regain a healthy relationship with food? How do we remove the emotional component of eating from our lives? It begins with a decision, and when you decide that your health and your weight is more important than some momentary food pleasure, you will have more incentive to shop for only healthy meats, fruits and vegetables. If you keep yourself and your shopping cart out of the snack food aisle, you'll be doing yourself a big favor when you get a late night urge to munch and you only have some almonds—not peanut brittle—in the pantry.

Chapter 5

Tips, Tricks and Strategies

One of the things that helped us on this program was to remind ourselves that we can do anything for a few weeks. That is one of the benefits of this program—it is only for a short time. Those foods that you like are not going anywhere. They will still be available when and if you are ready to have them again. It also helped us to remind ourselvs what a transient pleasure eating rich foods can be. They may taste good on the moment, but later you may feel a whole host of negative emotions, such as guilt, disappointment, and regret. Rich foods may also cause physical discomfort, such as feeling bloated, having clothes that feel too tight around your stomach, becoming tired, and experiencing weight gain.

It also helped us to think about the motto that Kate Moss, the model, said she lives by which is, "Nothing tastes as good as being thin feels." As you lose weight on this program, it becomes easier and easier to stick to it. Reminding ourselves that if we blow it, then we will set ourselves back for three days also gave us a lot of incentive to stay on track.

You can make it easier for yourself by preparing your meals ahead of time. When we were broiling chicken or steak, we would broil enough for the next few days. This way at lunch or dinner we were able to quickly get our meal together. While this program requires commitment and attention to detail, you can make your meals fairly quickly and easily if you decide to.

The Daily Weigh-In

An important part of this program is weighing yourself daily. It is good to have an accurate scale you can use. The effectiveness of daily weighing was confirmed in a study, conducted by researchers at Brown University. They found that people who weighed themselves every day were less likely to regain lost weight than were those who weighed themselves less often. It is easy to kid ourselves when we stop looking at the scale.

It is a mistake to believe that you will be able to tell if you gain weight by seeing if your clothes become too tight after doing the HCG program. The reason for this is that Dr. Simeons found that after a course of HCG, as much as ten pounds can be regained without any noticeable change in how your clothes fit you. This is due to the fact that at first any newly acquired fat is evenly distributed and does not show a preference for certain parts of your body as it did before.

Eating Out

Although it is important to be careful when eating out on the low calorie phase of the HCG program, we have found that there are some good options. You can look up the nutrition values of most restaurants online.

You can order a grilled steak salad with balsamic vinegar on the side. You will want to eat just the steak and the greens. Do your best to estimate the 3.5 ounces of steak and take the rest home.

Even Arby's and other fast food places offer a chicken breast option that will work. Enjoy with a side of green beans and you will be satisfied and well within the program guidelines. Estimate the 100 grams (3.5 ounces) of chicken and take the rest home.

A shrimp cocktail is always a winner and can be ordered at many restaurants. You can squeeze some lemon on your shrimp and perhaps either eliminate the cocktail sauce or just put one drop on each piece of shrimp. Most shrimp cocktails have less than 100 grams of shrimp. It's a good idea to have a small container of sauce with you, such as Walden Farms no-calorie barbecue sauce, when eating out.

If you are concerned that you went over your calorie limit by eating out, then you can always make it up by skipping your breadstick or piece of melba toast.

Your New Wardrobe

After completing the program and losing weight, it is a good idea to go through your clothes. Now you can enjoy fitting into those clothes you have been holding on to and hoping that someday you would be able to wear them again. You may wish to go shopping and buy some new clothes that look good on you and fit your new, slimmer body. Consider giving away some of those clothes that are now too big for you. This way someone else can enjoy them and you can feel added incentive to retain your new figure as you will not have those big clothes to go back to.

Your Eating Identities

In his book, "Healing and Recovery", Dr. David Hawkins discusses Dr. Eric Berne, author of "Games People Play", and others in the transactional analysis field. They explained how we all have three tapes we play over and over to ourselves that are like three voices in our head. They represent the "child", the "adult" and the "parent". When we sit down to eat, it is frequently the child who shows up. Since a child does not know anything about dieting and is often interested in immediate gratification, we sometimes eat too much and consume all of the wrong foods when we allow the child in us to be in charge. Of course, when the meal is over the child leaves and is replaced by the voice of the parent. This sounds something like this, "How could you have eaten all of that? What were you thinking? What is wrong with you?" Throughout this process the adult within us has disappeared.

According to Dr. Hawkins, we can start to combat this process simply by being aware of it. We can call forth the adult within us at mealtime and not allow our inner child to take over. Since we do not overindulge when under the influence of the adult, the adult remains with us and the parent does not need to show up when the meal has been completed. Thus, we have broken this unhealthy pattern. Dr. Hawkins recommends putting a sign on your refrigerator that says, "Adults only". Whatever helps you to be more aware of this process will help you to overcome it. We have found that since the HCG takes away much of your appetite, it makes it easier to keep the adult with you at mealtimes.

Doing this program has helped us to understand that there are many psychological reasons why we eat. When you find that most of your appetite has been taken away and yet you still want to eat, you begin to realize that a lot of why we eat has nothing to do with being hungry.

Better with a Buddy

It can also be helpful to do the program with a close friend or family member. We did the program together and it has been really wonderful for us both. We were able to prepare the same meal and we encouraged and supported each other. We cheered each other's results and helped each other to stay on track. We also did not tempt each other to go out to dinner, but rather did our best to find other ways, such as going to the movies, reading a good book, and shopping for new clothes, to relax and have fun.

We have known of many others who have done this program successfully together, too. Often one spouse may do it, and then the other, seeing their great results, gets on board. That is what happened to me (Felicia) when I saw how well Tony was doing with it. The same is true of friends and family members. We are always amazed at how many people have learned about this HCG program from a friend, family member or co-worker. As they say, "Seeing is believing". While this program may sound strange at first and you might find yourself wondering if you can do it, seeing the dramatic positive results others have achieved can definitely help you believe you can do it, too.

Pre-existing Health Conditions

If you have any health conditions, such as high blood pressure or the stable type of diabetes, then it is a good idea to monitor your blood pressure or blood sugar while on this program. As you lose weight, you are very likely to improve with these conditions and may require less medication than you are currently taking. Dr. Simeons often found that after the first few days of the low calorie diet with the HCG that his patients no longer needed their anti-diabetic medication, even when they had suffered from their condition for several years.

Dr. Simeons noticed that when his patients had a normal amount of circulating cholesterol before they began the HCG program that this tended to neither increase or decrease. However, when an obese patient with abnormally high cholesterol, who already showed signs of arteriosclerosis, did the HCG program, then their cholesterol would sometimes soar. Although this alarmed him at first, he found that no harm came to them and in the months following the HCG program their cholesterol levels tended to return to their pre-HCG program levels. We recommend that you always consult with your doctor about any health questions, medications, or concerns, especially if you have medical conditions that are weight-related. This cannot be stressed or said often enough.

Self-Talk

It is a good idea to pay attention to the things you tell yourself. Some people say, "I need to lose weight." It is good to put this in the present and to make it more active and positive. "I am losing weight" seems to work well, as does, "I am making positive changes in my life" or anything along these lines. Focus on the outcome you are desiring, rather than on what you feel you have to do, but do not really want to.

Years ago when I (Felicia) wanted to lose weight, I found myself frequently saying, "I want to lose weight." However, the scale did not budge. One day it occurred to me that saying I wanted to lose weight just kept me experiencing this wanting. That day I began to tell myself, "I am losing weight." I then found that I was able to change my eating habits and was able to lose the weight I desired.

Homeopathic Instructions

If you are using the homeopathic HCG drops, then it is important that you do not let the dropper touch your mouth. If you do, then do not put it back in the bottle.

Do not expose your bottle to x-rays.

Store your HCG drops in a cool dry place. If you do this and keep your bottle sealed, then it will last indefinitely.

Take the drops between meals, on an empty stomach. Wait at least 30 minutes before eating or drinking.

Be sure to take the recommended number of drops the suggested number of times each day. It would be very difficult to have just 500 calories/day and be comfortable if it were not for the HCG helping you to access your fat stores. In this way, you are really living on the 500 calories plus your fat stores, which allows you to do this program comfortably.

Chapter 6

Loading Days (Phase 1) Recipes

Most people look forward to enjoying their favorite "guilty pleasures" without the guilt on loading days. Don't be shy, this is your opportunity to give your body a good helping of fat in your system. Because the HCG is also in your system, you will not really eat as much as you imagine, and you may even need to force it. Here are some fun recipes to get your imagination started.

Apple Pie Overload

- apple pie
- pint of ice cream
- whipped cream

Cut pie into thirds, add 1/3 pint of ice cream. Top with whipped cream. Enjoy!

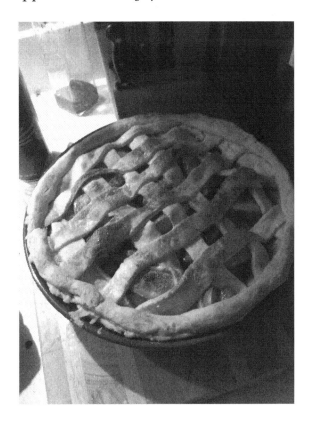

Nut Butter Gorge

- nut butter
- tablespoon or fingers

Enjoy!

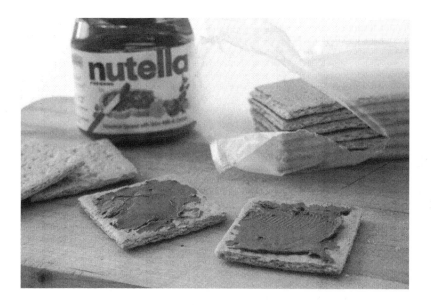

Extra Heavy Frappe

- half cup, ice cream
- 2 Tbsp, heavy cream
- $\frac{1}{4}$ c., milk

Mix ingredients in a blender. Enjoy!

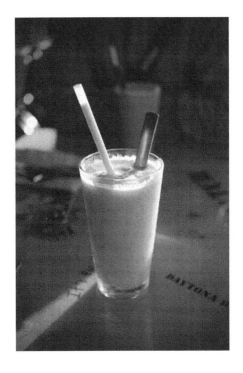

Ice Cream Madness

- 4 scoops of your favorite ice cream
- chocolate syrup

You know what to do... Enjoy!

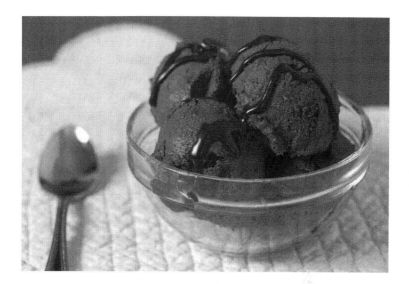

No Holds Barred Dessert

- 1 piece chocolate cake
- 1 scoop ice cream
- 2 Tbsp whipped cream

1. Find a heavy, rich piece of chocolate cake.
2. Add a scoop of your favorite ice cream.
3. Optionally top with whipped cream.

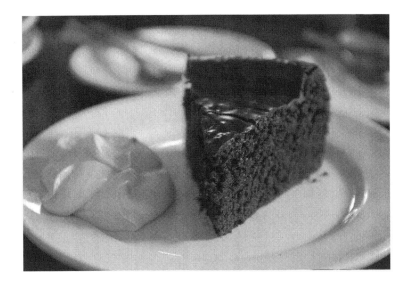

Pizza for One

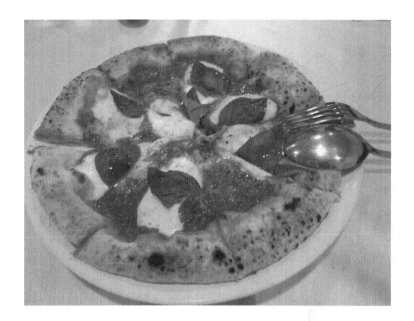

Chapter 7

HCG Very-Low-Calorie Diet (Phase 2) Recipes

There is no need to be hungry during this phase. While the HCG takes care of the physical hunger, sometimes you just want to drink or nosh on something extra.

If you would like something sweet, then you can have some green tea or other herbal tea with stevia or some other natural sweetener. You can also enjoy a coffee frappe, with coffee, ice and stevia.

Sugar-free Coffee Frappe

- 1 package, instant coffee (decaf or caffeinated)
- 4 drops, stevia
- 8 cubes, ice

1. Pour coffee/stevia mixture in a blender
2. Blend at a medium speed until ice is all crushed
3. Pour into a cup and serve
4. You may wish to stir with a spoon as you drink it so that it doesn't separate

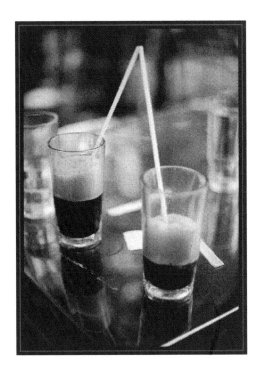

Lo-Cal Strawberry Smoothie

- 5 frozen strawberries
- 8 oz, water or iced tea
- 1 tbsp, lemon juice
- 4 drops, stevia

1. Pour strawberries, liquid, and stevia in a blender
2. Blend at a medium speed until the strawberries form a slush
3. Pour into a cup and serve
4. Enjoy with a spoon or a straw

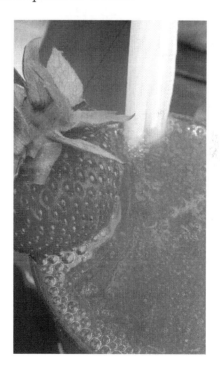

Chunky Beef Stew

- 100 grams (3.5 ounces), lean beef cuts
- ⅓ cup, water
- 1 can, diced tomatoes
- 1 tsp, chili powder
- 1 tsp, onion powder
1. Braise meat in a skillet for 30 minutes.

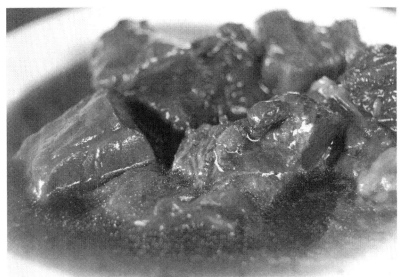

Beefy Tomato Chili

- 100 grams (3.5 ounces), lean beef cuts
- 1 can, tomato paste
- 1 can, diced tomatoes
- 1 tsp, chili powder
- 1 tsp, onion powder

1. Braise meat in a skillet for 20 minutes.

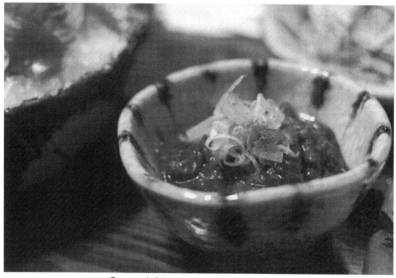

Broiled Scallops

- 100 grams (3.5 ounces), scallops
- 6, cherry tomatoes
- 2 tbsp, lemon juice
- 1 clove, garlic

1. Broil fish in the oven for 10 minutes until cooked tender and flaky.
2. Squeeze fresh lemon juice over the fish and tomatoes
3. Enjoy!

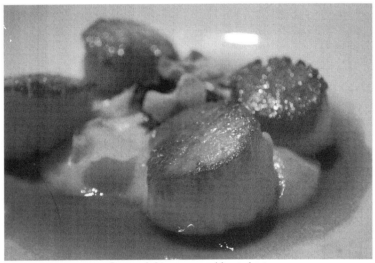

Spicy Grilled Tilapia

- 100 grams (3.5 ounces), tilapia or whitefish
- 4 stalks, asparagus
- 2 tbsp, lemon juice
- 1 tsp, chili powder
- 1 tsp, onion powder
- pinch, garlic

1. Arrange asapragus around fish in a baking pan
2. Sprinkle spices over food
3. Broil fish and asparagus in the oven for 10 minutes until fish is cooked white and flaky.

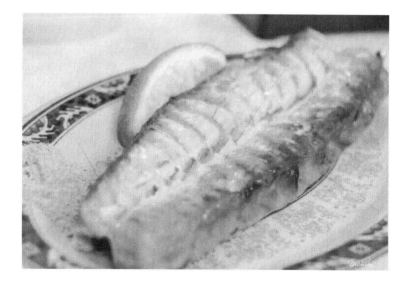

BBQ Chicken

- 100 grams (3.5 ounces), white meat chicken
- 1 can, 6 oz, tomato paste
- 3 tbsp, vinegar
- 1 tsp, lemon juice
- 12 drops, stevia
- pinch, garlic powder

1. Grill chicken until cooked.
2. Mix tomato paste, vinegar, lemon juice and stevia in a bowl.
3. Add oregano and garlic powder to taste.
4. Smear the chicken with the sauce mix.
5. Enjoy!

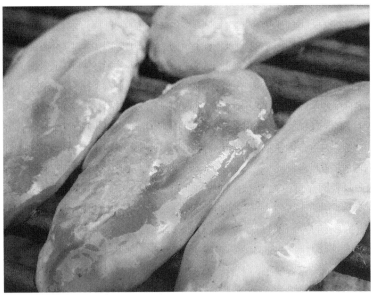

Baked Apple "Pie"

- 1 cored, apple
- 1 crumbled, bread stick
- 4 drops, stevia
- 1 pinch, cinnamon

1. arrange apple slices on crumbled bread stick on a microwave-safe plate
2. bake apple slices for 30 seconds in a microwave oven
3. sprinkle stevia and cinnamon on top

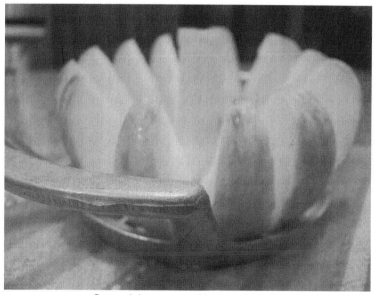

Chapter 8

Transition (Phase 3) Recipes

This phase is the start to "eating right for the rest of your life." Some will recognize the high-protein, low-carb elements of this as similar to the "Atkins diet." If you like cheese, eggs, and nuts you will enjoy the transition phase.

In this phase you can eat whatever you would like as long as you avoid sugars and starches. This means that you want to put away those breadsticks, apples and melba toast. Now you can enjoy things like eggs, cheese, nuts, hamburgers, dark meat chicken, all kinds of fish and heavy cream. You are no longer limited to just 3.5 ounces of protein at a meal, so you can enjoy that big, juicy steak if you would like. You are also able to cook with oils and butter, since these are not a problem as you are not eating starches. You can enjoy a coffee frappe with heavy cream and sugar-free, carbohydrate-free whipped cream on top. Or, you can indulge in a strawberry smoothie, also with heavy cream and whipped cream made with heavy cream and stevia.

Creamy Coffee Frappe

- 1 serving of instant coffee (decaf or caffeinated)
- 4 drops of stevia
- 8 ice cubes
- 3 Tbsp heavy cream

1. Pour in the coffee/stevia/ice/ heavy cream mixture into blender
2. Blend in the blender
3. Pour into a cup and serve
4. You can add sugar-free, carb-free whipped cream. (Find at certain grocery stores, such as Wal-Mart, or please see whipped cream recipe.)

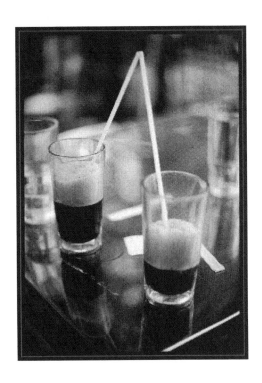

Cheesy Gooey Omelette

- 3 eggs
- ½ cup, grated cheddar cheese
- 1 Tbsp heavy cream

1. beat eggs in a bowl until yolks are mixed
2. add heavy cream
3. pour into hot, lightly greased, skillet
4. cook until firm
5. flip over and pour cheese onto egg
6. cover, cook for 1 minute

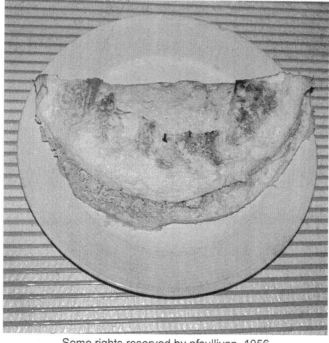

Creamy Strawberry Smoothie

- 5 frozen strawberries
- 4 drops of stevia
- 4 oz of half and half
- 3 Tbsp heavy cream

1. Pour in the coffee/stevia/heavy cream mixture into blender
2. Blend in the blender
3. Pour into a cup and serve
4. You can add sugar-free, carb-free whipped cream. (Find at certain grocery stores, such as Wal-Mart, or please see whipped cream recipe.)

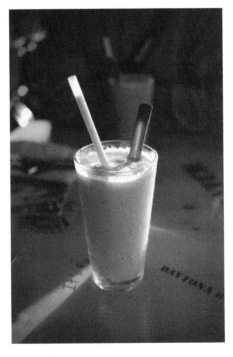

Chapter 9

Frequently Asked Questions

Why are eggs not allowed?

According to Dr. Simeons. although two good-sized eggs are equivalent to about 100 grams of meat, the yolk contains a large amount of fat. If a person were to develop an aversion to meat, then they could add the white of three eggs to one whole egg as a replacement. However, it is best to avoid having eggs to replace your meat unless you absolutely have to.

Are any cheeses allowed?

You can occasionally have 100 grams of cottage cheese, but only if it is made from skimmed milk. No other cheeses are allowed.

Would a large-frame, hard-working, muscular male eat the same amount as a small, elderly woman?

According to Dr. Simeons the answer is "yes". This is because under the effect of HCG the obese body is always able to get all the calories it needs from the abnormal fat deposits, regardless of whether it uses up 1500 calories or 4000 calories/day. Dr. Simeons also found that he was able to give both the large, muscular man and the small, elderly woman the same amount of HCG.

Can I make substitutions in the program as long as they still add up to 500 calories/day?

Dr. Simeons says you cannot and that it is very important to stick with the way the program is written. For example, you cannot substitute an extra breadstick for an apple. Although you are not adding extra calories, this is likely to prevent you from losing weight. It is important to remember that Dr. Simeons researched this extensively on thousands of patients. Therefore, it is best to do this program accurately and to remember that it is just for a few weeks.

What is the composition of the 500 calories?

The daily ration should consist of 200 grams (7 ounces) of fat-free protein and a very small amount of starch. The remainder of the calories come mostly from fruits and vegetables.

What should strict vegetarians do?

They must replace the animal protein by drinking 500 cc. of skimmed milk/day, though part of this ration can be consumed with curds. The fruit, vegetables and breadsticks or melba toast remain the same. Even so, a vegetarian will generally lose only about half of what a non-vegetarian will lose, presumably due to the sugar content of the milk. Vegetarians may therefore find that this program may not be for them.

Will my body lose the vitamins and minerals by losing weight so quickly?

According to Dr. Simeons, when a person loses a pound of fatty tissue, which they do almost daily while on the program, only the actual fat is burned up. All the vitamins, the proteins, the blood and the minerals that this tissue contains are fed back into the body. He further stated that a low blood count that is not due to any serious disorder of the blood-forming tissues tends to improve on the program. In addition, he never encountered a significant protein deficiency nor signs of a lack of vitamins in any of the thousands of patients he worked with, who were dieting regularly.

Can I take my usual supplements while on the program?

We have found with the homeopathic HCG drops that a person can take their usual supplements except for fish oil (due to its fat content). Of course, it is a good idea to read your labels and to avoid any supplements that contain sugar, carbohydrates or fats as these will interfere with your weight loss. The scale, too, will always be your best guide. If you take a supplement and your weight increases the next day, then it would be best to refrain from this supplement while on the program. Personally, we have not found Vitamin C,

Vitamin B12, Vitamin D-3, multi-minerals or silica gel to interfere with the homeopathic HCG drops. In fact, Dr. Simeons did allow calcium and Vitamin D, although not in an oily solution if he had a patient whose teeth were in poor condition. He also permitted Vitamin C in large doses with an antihistamine at the onset of a common cold. He also found that it was fine to use an antibiotic if it was required, for instance by the dentist. He even allowed cortisone during treatment in cases of bronchial asthma and hay fever. Of course, it is a good idea to consult your doctor if you require medications.

What happens if I eat something like a brownie that is not on the program?

Dr. Simeons said that if a person eats something that is not on the list of allowed foods that they can expect to lose about three days of progress on their program. In this case, it is best not to kick yourself and to just continue with the program. Personally, we have found knowing this to provide us with added incentive to be meticulous about eating only what is allowed.

Why is it important to eat to capacity lots of fatty and sugary foods on the two loading days?

Dr. Simeons found that the people who did this correctly tended to feel remarkably well while on the program, whereas those who did not often did not feel as light, clear-headed and comfortable until being on the program for about a week and a half.

Do the loading days have any other benefits besides expanding a person's fat cells so that they can lose weight more quickly?

Many people report that on loading days, the joy of being able to eat whatever they wanted is met with surprise that they cannot get all the food down. They often feel full to capacity and are excited to begin the low-calorie part of the diet. We have had this experience ourselves. Psychologically, it seems that people often realize that gluttonously eating any food they desire is not all that they thought it would be. Part of it seems to be that the HCG takes away so much of a person's appetite that they do not experience the enjoyment that they imagined. As a result, these two loading days seem to take away much of the desire for fatty and sugary foods. Although this is not the reason for doing these two loading days, this appears to be an added benefit of doing this program.

Will my weight come off steadily or are there fluctuations in how rapidly I lose weight?

Dr. Simeons found that people usually gained a few pounds during their two loading days. Then usually within the first 48 hours, they lost all of this weight and sometimes more. For the next few days they often continue to lose as much as two pounds a day. After the fourth or fifth day of the low calorie phase, the daily weight loss often slows to about a pound or less per day. Men then tend to lose pretty steadily at this rate, although women may be more irregular, sometimes not losing anything for two or three days and then experiencing a loss of a few pounds. He felt this was due to women experiencing more variations in their retention and elimination of water.

We have found that how rapidly a person loses weight seems to depend on a number of factors such as how well they did their loading days, how much weight they have to lose, and how well they follow the program. We know of one woman who weighed over 300 pounds. She lost 35 pounds during her first ten days on the low calorie part of the program before her weight loss slowed down. However, this is quite rare, was probably mostly water weight and certainly is not typical.

Are there other reasons that I may not lose weight (or even gain weight) while on this program?

Dr. Simeons found that on or about the day of ovulation or during the three days preceding menstruation that some women might gain a little weight or might not lose weight. He felt it was best to ignore this as the weight loss resumed once these events had passed.

He found that sometimes a person who thought they were doing the program correctly, but who was not losing or even gaining weight were often committing some type of error. In this case it is important to immediately figure out the reason for this. Dr. Simeons noticed that the slightest increase in calories from a salted almond, a glass of tomato juice, a few potato chips, etc., resulted in an increase in weight the following day. He explained that the reason for this is that under the influence of the HCG the blood is saturated with food and the blood volume can only just accommodate the 500 calories. Any extra calories force the blood to increase its volume sufficiently to hold the extra food. Therefore, it is not the weight of the extra food, but rather the amount of water the body must retain to accommodate this food that often leads to weight gain. Once a person has stopped the HCG, their blood is no longer saturated and they can easily accommodate extra food without having to increase its volume. Thus, it is a very sensitive program that one must follow to the best of their ability to obtain the best results.

Should I limit my salt intake while on this program?

According to Dr. Simeons, there is no restriction in a person's intake of salt. However, it is important that a person drink plenty of water (about 2 liters) while on this program. Although a person can use salt freely, Dr. Simeons felt that the daily amount consumed should remain about the same as a sudden increase in salt will result in an increase in weight from one day to the next. However, this type of weight gain can be ignored as it can be accounted for as being due to an increase in salt intake from the previous day.

What happens if I don't drink enough water?

Dr. Simeons explained that the amount of water a person retains has nothing to do with the amount of water they drink. If their fluid intake is insufficient to meet their body's requirements, then it will withhold water from the kidneys and they will notice less frequent and highly concentrated urine output, putting a strain on their kidneys. However, if a person drinks too much water, then the surplus is quickly and easily eliminated and so it is better to err in this direction.

Will I be constipated on the low calorie part of this program?

Dr. Simeons noted that obese people frequently suffer from constipation. Drinking lots of water does help. He found that it was normal for people to have a bowel movement every three or four days while on the program due to the restricted nature of their diet. However, he never permitted his patients to use any kind of laxative taken by mouth while on the program. Only if four days had passed without a bowel movement and they were bothered by this, would he allow them to use a suppository. Once the low calorie part of the diet had ended, people tended to find their bowel movements would return to normal.

We have found with the homeopathic HCG drops that herbal tea that contains Senna, such as Uncle Lee's Dieter's Tea, can be taken without interfering with the diet. It is important to start slowly by steeping your tea no more than two minutes in the evening to start with. If you do not have the desired result the next morning, then you can increase to three minutes that night and so on. If the result is more than you desire, then it is best to steep your tea bag for less time. This is very powerful tea and should be used carefully.

Are there other reasons for not losing weight or even gaining weight on the program?

Sometimes this can be the result of absentmindedly tasting the food one is cooking, having a slightly bigger portion than is allowed, forgetting one has already had their second breadstick or apple, etc. Dr. Simeons found that if people carefully reviewed their eating, then they would frequently realize the error they had made.

When no dietary error appeared to have been made, then Dr. Simeons would focus on a person's use of cosmetics. He found that fats, oils, creams and ointments are absorbed in the skin and that they would interfere with a person's weight reduction while on the HCG. This is true even for people who regularly handle fats, such as butchers, massage therapists, hair stylists, etc. In fact, he had one man who had a glass eye, who realized that the ointment he would put in his eyesocket interfered with his weight loss. Once he stopped using it, his regular weight loss resumed. The HCG program really is that sensitive.

Dr. Simeons found that while on the HCG normal fat is restored to the skin, making it appear much more youthful. Therefore, it is not as hard to go without ones usual lotions and creams as you might think while on the program. Of course, it is good to avoid being in the sun or to cover oneself with a hat, long sleeves and/or pants if sun exposure cannot be avoided while on the program.

Are there any other things I should look out for to avoid sabotaging my weight loss while on the program?

Dr. Simeons cautioned a person about unwittingly taking chewing gum, throat lozenges, certain vitamin pills, cough syrups, etc., that contain sugar or fats as this may interfere with their regular loss of weight. Of course, here, too, your scale can also be your guide.

We found that it is better to avoid things like chewing gum. Although you can buy sugar-free gum, it may contain carbohydrates and would thus interfere with your weight loss. In fact, we found that some sugarless gum actually contains two carbohydrates per piece. This can really trip you up and prevent you from losing weight on the low calorie part of this program, as well as when you are in transition. Also, be careful with cough drops or cough syrup. Reading labels is always a good thing to do.

The only self-medication that Dr. Simeons allowed was an aspirin for a headache. He noted that some people did experience a slight headache during the first week of treatment, especially if they did not do their loading properly. However, he found that after about a week, this would usually disappear. He also permitted oral contraceptives.

How will I sleep while on the program?

Dr. Simeons found that a lot of people did not require as much sleep while doing the low calorie part of the program. We have found that people often have a lot of energy since they are accessing their fat stores and not just living off of the 500 calories/day. Therefore, people often feel surprisingly good during this phase. Personally, we have found that we sleep well on the program, though we do not seem to need as much sleep.

Can I get a massage while on the HCG program?

According to Dr. Simeons, it is better not to have a massage during the low calorie phase. He found it is better for people not to disturb their body's adjusting itself to their rapid loss of fat and that it is better for them to wait until after they have completed the program before getting a massage. In addition, the fats in the lotions and oils a massage therapist uses are a problem for someone on the low calorie phase as they will be absorbed by the skin and interfere with their weight loss.

Is it possible for me to go below my ideal weight with the HCG program?

When a person no longer has any abnormal fat to be put into circulation, then Dr. Simeons found that people would feel a sudden, constant hunger. In addition, their body would start to consume normal fat and he found that this was always regained once they resumed normal eating. As a result, Dr. Simeons did not find that a person could go below their normal weight with the HCG program.

Will I be comfortable eating a 500-calorie/day diet?

Dr. Simeons found that although many people were skeptical that they could be comfortable on this program, they were often able to overcome their doubts by talking with others, who had done the program. We have noticed that many people are nervous about eating only 500 calories/day and then are pleasantly surprised that it is not as difficult as they thought it would be. Often it is by seeing others' results and learning about their experiences that people are able to overcome their doubts and give this a try. We have found that over 99% of the more than 1,000 people we know who have tried this have been able to be successful with it, as long as they have done it correctly. It seems to be the people who have not tried it, who are concerned that it will be difficult and not work. Personally, we have had great success with this program ourselves and have seen so many others also achieve their weight loss goals that we are convinced of the program's efficacy and value. In fact, we have never found any diet that has been so rapid and effective. We feel that Dr. Simeons' groundbreaking work is of great benefit and, like him, believe that the HCG can help just about anyone achieve their weight loss goals.

Will I keep my weight off in the transition phase if I eat fairly normally and just avoid sugar and starch?

Yes. In fact, Dr. Simeons found that people who tried to continue with the 500 calories/day during this phase found themselves feeling extremely hungry and actually gained weight. This is due to their body retaining water since they experienced a protein deficiency at this low caloric intake without the HCG. Therefore, it is best to return to eating a normal caloric amount while simply avoiding sugar and starch during this phase. When Dr. Simeons encountered a patient who had attempted to continue with the 500 calories/day during this transition phase and had been stunned to find themselves gaining weight, he would have them eat two eggs for breakfast, a huge steak for lunch and dinner followed by a large helping of cheese. Most of the time, these patients would find that the next day they had lost about two pounds and that they had passed large quantities of water.

How likely am I to keep my weight off after completing the HCG and transition phases?

Dr. Simeons found that 60-70% of his patients had little or no difficulty keeping their weight off permanently. He found that the ones who did regain some of their weight had stopped weighing themselves daily. He felt that daily weighing is essential since a person can easily gain ten pounds without noticing a difference in their clothing after a course of HCG. The reason for this is that after you have completed the HCG program and transition phases, newly acquired fat is evenly distributed at first and therefore does not have its former preference to attach itself to certain parts of the body.

In addition, Dr. Simeons found that older teenage girls, who have previously experienced bouts of compulsive overeating, tend to have the worst relapse rates. Women who have done the HCG program at the onset of menopause (within one year of having their last menstruation) also have a higher rate of relapse until their menopause is well-established.

According to Dr. Simeons, people who have done the HCG program once seem to do even better on additional rounds since they now know how to do the diet and that they can do it comfortably and successfully.

Is there any muscular fatigue doing this program?

As a person approaches the end of the low-calorie phase, when they have lost a lot of weight quite rapidly, Dr. Simeons sometimes found that they would feel like it was more difficult than usual to lift something heavy or climb a set of stairs. It is not that they become short of breath or feel exhausted. It is just that they may feel that their muscles have to work harder to accomplish this task. Dr. Simeons noticed that this feeling would disappear soon after they had stopped taking the HCG. He explained that it is caused by the removal of abnormal fat in and around the muscles. This makes the muscles too long, causing them to have to perform a greater contraction than before when bending an arm, etc. He found that within a short time the muscles have adjusted themselves to their new situation and everything feels fine again. Dr. Simeons discovered that this phenomenon was less likely to occur in people who continued to exercise regularly while doing the HCG program.

Should I be exercising while on this program?

Surprisingly, Dr. Simeons found that a person's weight might actually increase on this program if they exercise strenuously for a long period of time to the point of exhaustion. Unless the person is in great shape, then a long walk or run, a day of skiing, rowing, bicycling or even dancing can result in weight gain on the following day. He did not find this be the case after a game of tennis, a vigorous swim, a short run, a ride on horseback or a game of golf. Although additional calories are consumed by the extra muscular effort involved in strenuous physical activity, it appears to be offset by the retention of water that the tired circulation cannot immediately eliminate. Therefore, it is better while on the low-calorie part of this program not to engage in strenuous exercise.

This can be of great benefit to people, who are very overweight in that it enables them to lose the weight before they resume exercising. It reminds us of the following joke: "My doctor told me I shouldn't work out until I'm in better shape. I told him, 'All right; don't send me a bill until I pay you.'" – Comedian Steven Wright

When a person is very overweight, it can be difficult to exercise. The extra stress on their knees and joints, as well as the extra pounds they have to carry around with them can be a great impediment to a physical workout. Did you know that your knees bear the brunt of your body weight? In fact, every extra pound you carry adds up to 3 pounds of pressure on your knee joints when you walk and 10 pounds when you run. It is no wonder that overweight people frequently have knee problems. This, of course, makes exercising even more difficult until the weight has been lost. After someone has done the HCG program and has lost much of their excess weight, then they are in better shape to exercise comfortably.

Chapter 10

Sharing HCG Diet Experiences

We wanted to share our experiences on the HCG diet, as well as the experiences of others we have known. What has impressed us is that this program works well for both men and women, as well as people of all ages. We have known several women who have gained a lot of weight during their pregnancy, who have found this program to be especially helpful in losing those unwanted pounds. We've also been impressed with how well older people have done on this program. It seems to especially work well for people who have physical conditions that make it difficult for them to exercise.

Felicia's experience:

For the past few years, I have been thinking that I would like to lose 10 pounds. Then I learned about HCG or Human Chorionic Gonadotrophin hormone. What was impressive about Dr. Simeons' work was that people were able to lose weight in all the right places, while not feeling extreme hunger. Although a 500-calorie diet without HCG would require an enormous amount of will power to achieve and would not be a healthy way to lose weight, he found that adding HCG changed all this. Fortunately, I learned that HCG is now available in homeopathic form, making it very inexpensive and allowing people to easily administer themselves. Having been a firm believer in homeopathy for many years, I was curious to see how this worked. I have to admit, however, that the 500 calories/day made me hesitant to begin this plan. My husband Tony, however, did not have these reservations and he decided to give it a try. He found that the HCG drops took away most of his hunger and that 500-calories left him feeling satisfied. He has now completed 3 rounds of the diet and has lost 40 pounds. Finally, on his last round, he persuaded me to try it. It was not as difficult as it sounded. I especially enjoyed the first two "loading" days, where you are told to eat lots of fatty and sugary foods in order to expand your fat cells and make it easier for your body to access them. I kept reminding myself that I can do anything for a few weeks. After 26 days, I had happily lost over 11 pounds. I also lost inches in all the right places and not where I did not want to lose them. In addition, I no longer have some of the aches and pains that I used to have. I marveled at how many of us go through years of wanting to lose weight, but not taking the positive steps necessary to achieve our goal. Weighing what I weighed almost thirty years ago when I was in my early twenties has been a wonderful accomplishment for me and it all occurred very quickly. I hope those of you wanting to lose weight will not wait another day to look and feel the way you would like. It is definitely worth it.

Tony's experience:

A few years ago, my weight was spiraling out of control. I was going to the gym and eating only about 900 calories/day and was still not losing weight. In fact, if I missed a day at the gym or ate a little more, then I would even gain more weight. I was very discouraged and just about ready to give up what felt like a losing battle, when I discovered the HCG program. I have now done the HCG protocol several times and have lost a total of 40 pounds. Most importantly, I weigh what I did in high school over 30 years ago and I feel great! My knees and feet no longer ache and I have more energy for my life. The HCG protocol has eliminated the bad cravings and habits I had around food. I have tracked my weight steadily for the past 18 months and this habit alone has helped make my weight loss permanent. I can't fool myself: the scale never lies!

Here are the experiences of some of the people we have known:

I am a mother of 2 young boys ages 3 and 1.
Before I had my first child I was in a size 8 -

10. After I gave birth, I was in a size 16. And after I had my second child I was a size 18. I tried other diets while exercising and would not lose much weight. I decided to try the HCG diet because I needed to keep up with my boys. Also, I had little time to exercise while dieting. This protocol provided me a solution.

I like this diet so much for the fact that it's easy and I had instant gratification. Morning after morning, I saw less pounds and/or inches. I never felt hungry on this diet. I prepared all my food for the week on Sundays; therefore, my meals were always ready when it was time for me to eat. And I didn't have to worry about cooking a meal for my family and a meal for myself every night.

I thought participating in special occasions, like award shows, birthday parties, the pumpkin patch, etc. would cause a problem for me. I found there was always a solution. I would either munch on an apple, pass on the food, or I would go to the chef personally and tell him to make me a shrimp soup with spinach, no sugar, oil, and starches. I would make this soup at home as well. It is so fulfilling! Again, I was never hungry on this diet.

Now, that I am at the end of the very low calorie diet, I have lost over 26 pounds in 38 days. I feel wonderful, have more energy, and I am still not hungry. I can now run in the park with my boys. I am looking forward to shopping for new clothes. If I can do it with 2 little boys and a husband to keep up with, anyone can.
—Y.G.

I weighed 150 lbs. when I started the HCG diet and now I weigh 133 lbs. I wore size 10 pants and now I wear size 6. I lost the weight without having to go to the gym. I eat healthier and make better choices when I go out to eat. Weighing myself daily helped me see what made me gain weight. I gain weight when I eat bread and other food that has wheat in it. If I eat it then I know I will weigh a little more the next day. I had tried other diets but they didn't work. I lost 6 lbs on one diet but then I gained it back. Felicia and Tony have been helpful with answering any questions that I have about the drops and the diet.
—M.D.

When I first heard about HCG, I did not think I could sustain myself on the 500-calorie diet required to do the program. After seeing the incredible weight loss my two friends attained through the diet, I decided it was worth trying. I found the diet combined with the HCG the most effortless and quickest way I have ever lost weight. I lost 24 pounds in 23 days and have never felt better. Since HCG combined with the required diet works as a detox for your body, I not only lost weight, but I felt both physically and mentally better. I have been dealing with anxiety most of my adult life and I have noticed an immense improvement in my mental well being.
—N.H.

I love the HCG and have lost 38 pounds. I have my husband on it and he has lost 20 pounds. People I work with see how much I have lost and they are getting on it, too. I can get into clothes that I had 20 years ago. I have also gotten compliments on how good I look and have given your web site out to several people all over.
—R.M.

The product is truly amazing! I am following it to the "T" and have lost 21 pounds in 22 days. A lot of what I'm losing is the pregnancy baby fat I had a hard time losing and gave up trying to lose. I gained over 60 lbs during my pregnancy; ate healthy, no candy, soda nor any cravings. Doctor said my body was like a weightlifter on steroids and hoarding things. He even took me off milk products. So I greatly appreciate your site.
—K.C.

When we saw Tony recently at the Wellness Expo, I asked him what he'd been doing to lose so much weight. He told me it was HCG. I knew about the product because my Mom, who lives out of state, has been doing HCG and keeping the weight off successfully. I was excited to learn that Tony and Felicia also sell the product through their company Shifting Frequencies. It was no coincidence to find a wonderful, source of HCG that we could trust. We're near the end of our first round and we've been thrilled with the fast and easy weight loss. My husband has lost over 25 pounds and I have lost close to 20 since we started about 22 days ago. HCG is the answer to our prayers!
—G.P.

I am 76 years old and I have tried many different diets over the years. Often I would lose some weight, however, I would then return to my old eating habits and would quickly gain it back. I felt that I was not just fat, but actually was obese. Last year I learned about the HCG diet program and decided to give it a try. Since the diet is basically a three week program (23 days with the first two being loading days), I felt it was worth a shot. As it turned out, I found the diet easy to do. The homeopathic HCG drops took away most of my appetite and there were days when I didn't even want to eat all the food that was allowed. The weight dropped off quickly and I was excited to find myself at a weight which I had not seen in over 20 years. I was able to wear clothes that I had not been able to fit into for many, many years and the pains in my knees and legs from my arthritis have lessened considerably. When I entered the transition phase, I was amazed at how easy it was to do. Even though I could eat a lot more food, I was still able to lose more weight. Since then I continue to weigh myself every day. Although I go out to dinner at least once a week and usually gain a pound or two, I am then careful for the next few days and am able to lose this weight. Approximately five months have passed since I started the HCG diet and not only have I kept the weight off, but I have even managed to lose another eight pounds. I have changed my eating habits dramatically and couldn't be happier.

—I.W.

If you are reading this, you are curious at least and possibly desperate to make a change. Perhaps you're thinking: "Yea, I know I can lose weight on some diet, but talk to me after 6 months or a year". Well, that's what I would like to do. First I need to toss my skinny jeans in the dryer.

I lost 23 pounds on the injection form in fall 2009. I hated the injections, but didn't know another way. I went off one short round just before Thanksgiving, did another and went off for Christmas. I gained a few pounds back, but essentially stabilized as 20 pounds off until the end of summer 2010. I knew I was over-eating, but blamed it on hormones or the inner rebellious child or simply a summer too hot to exercise and I gained 7 pounds back. Cravings were back. I tried Atkins, but the scale didn't budge.

One morning I knew I was ready to start a round again. I ordered the homeopathic form. I admit that I was skeptical: the protocol is hard enough with the real hormone, but honestly I didn't want to do the injections or go through the process to get it and mix it and inject it. Shifting Frequencies was wonderful to work with! I ordered online and my product arrived in a few days. Ready when I was ready. I knew the protocol worked, but the homeopathic formula was even more effective at curbing my hunger than the injections. I adjusted the drops for my body. I dropped the 7 pounds and a few more. My body told me it was time to end the round at 2 weeks. I've learned to honor that. This time, I've held within 3 pounds of my lowest weight.

Aside from the weight loss I eat what I want, however, what I want has changed. I really enjoy a great apple and a sirloin burger fried in a salted skillet with Dijon mustard over baby spinach! My tastes have changed along with my body. I love that I can really taste things and that while I do like a good cookie or whipped cream, I really don't like sweets or bread much at all. My cravings are rare and my portions are modest. I am free from fear that the 20 pounds will find me. I know that if a few do, I've got the protocol to end my cravings and restore balance in many areas of my life.

Since you're still reading, I will tell you what I tell anyone who is seriously thinking about this protocol. For me, the hardest part was thinking about how hard it was going to be. I exercise so I ate a little more of the allowed foods, but just a little. I found that I could not use artificial sweeteners of any kind, but that I could eat a BIG sweet juicy apple and still lose weight. I did best with lean beef and baby spinach. Your body will tell you want it needs. If you are an emotional eater, listen to what's going through your mind, how you talk to yourself about this process. It may be very insightful and if you are like me: Liberating.

The dryer's beeping but I'd better let those skinny jeans go a while longer. They are getting baggy!
—C.N.

It is always refreshing to receive service and smiles and information in one company. All of you have been so helpful.

When I first started using HCG, I had marched, kicking and screaming, right into morbid obesity. I followed "diets" and sought medical help to no avail. I was unable to stop the weight gain, even with lifestyle changes. The risks of diabetes had overtaken me. A nutritionalist had thrown the towel in on me when she suggested I try HCG. Let me tell you, HCG has altered my life.

Immediately I researched HCG (Human Chorionic Gonadotrophin hormone), read Dr. ATW Simeons book "Pounds and Inches", searched the internet, and I was encouraged that stored fat accumulation was what HCG targeted instead of muscle. The possibility of hunger suppression and body reshaping gave me the courage to attempt the 500 calorie a day regime.

I am thrilled to report I am 52 pounds lighter! Hope has been restored in a very, very disillusioned 67 year old woman. On a 4' 11" person, 52 pounds is enormous! I'm currently on my 4th round. I can honestly say I don't know which period I look forward to the most – the 28 days of losing weight or the 28 days of rest in which my weight stays the same on a good and healthy dietary schedule.

—L.L.T.

Chapter 11

The Upward Spiral

Usually people gain weight slowly over a long period of time. Due to the timeframe, they adjust to their greater and greater weight and hardly notice the tremendous stress this is placing on their body. We are always amazed at how heavy even one pound is. A five pound bag of flour, a ten pound bowling ball, etc. feels quite heavy. If you are forty pounds overweight, this is like walking around all day with four 10-pound bowling balls. If someone handed these to you and told you to carry them with you everywhere you go, it would be very difficult. Yet how many people cart around forty extra pounds all day, everyday without even realizing how much more challenging they are making things for themselves?

Each day on this program as the pounds and inches melt away people tend to find themselves feeling lighter, happier and full of energy. It is about being all that you can be- healthy, slim, attractively dressed, and feeling in charge of your life. Many people feel out of control with their weight. When you get back in control in one area of your life, then this can help you regain control in other areas as well. Also, by losing weight and reaching your goal, you can help to inspire others to achieve their desired weight as well.

Who inspires you?

Inspiring people help motivate us to expand our minds about what is possible. We remind ourselves that if they can do it, then so can we. We have always loved the statement in Lewis Carroll's "Alice in Wonderland" about believing 6 impossible things before breakfast.

About five years ago we were reading an article in the Journal of Longevity about Jack LaLanne, who is known as America's number one physical fitness expert. At that time he was 91-years-old and he still looked fantastic and was in incredible physical shape. Even at this age, he continued to work out two hours each day, 7 days a week, ate a nutritionally well-balanced diet of protein, fruits and vegetables, and he took about 40 to 50 supplements a day. More incredibly, he had not eaten any dessert since 1929!

We find his example of self-discipline and the fact that he said that he never thinks about age to be so inspiring. Research has shown that if people continue to exercise that they can maintain their muscular strength. Certainly Jack LaLanne is proof that this is true. He passed away at the age of 96 and will continue to inspire millions with his example of what is possible. One of our favorite sayings is, "Age is a matter of mind. If you don't mind, it doesn't matter". Jack LaLanne also helped all of us to expand our idea of what is possible. He helped us all to see that a person can remain vital, in great shape, and energetic throughout their life. You do not have to get old, become overweight, and experience weight-related health issues.

A few years back I (Felicia) was talking to my father and he said, "I think it is important in life to live up to one's potential". We both agree with him. We believe we all have enormous potential and that hard work and self-discipline do pay off. Our bodies are our vehicles and we encourage you to do all that you can to keep yours running in the best condition. There are many resources and people available to help you on your journey. We hope you will find what works best for you. Maybe you will become an inspiration to others and help show us all just how much is possible.

Researchers at the University of Texas-Austin found that on average,

> "Beautiful people are generally happier than their unattractive counterparts. Economists say it's largely because they get better jobs and marry successful people."

The economists analyzed data from five surveys conducted by social scientists in the U.S., Canada, Germany, and Britain. These surveys asked more than 25,000 thousand participants about their levels of happiness and also either required an interviewer to rate participants' attractiveness or evaluate their beauty from their pictures. The top 15 percent of people ranked by looks are over 10 percent happier than people ranked in the bottom 10 percent of looks, researchers say.

This research provides evidence for something that many people understand and believe- that society is biased in favor of more attractive people. Years ago Tony worked with a very heavy-set woman. He then left this job and we did not see her for a few years. When we did we were surprised to see that she had lost about 50 pounds and was actually now quite thin. She told us that she had lost her job and realized that since she was going to have to interview for a new job that she was more likely to be hired if she was thin. She therefore had lost the weight and she now had a new job she was happy with. While most of us do not wish to believe that people are biased in this way, research tends to support that it is true.

Several years ago, we heard best-selling author, Marianne Williamson, give a talk. She suggested that if a person is looking for their ideal mate that they make a list of all of the qualities they would like this person to have. Then she suggested they make a list of all of the qualities that this person would like to see in their mate. Finally, she encouraged them to work on being this person and then she felt that their ideal mate would show up. Often we are far more in control of our lives and the things that happen to us than we realize.

Marianne Williamson has also said, "Personal transformation can and does have global effects. As we go, so goes the world, for the world is us. The revolution that will save the world is ultimately a personal one." With obesity at an all-time high in the United States, we think it is fair to say that what most people have been doing has not been working. Maybe it is time to give something else a try.

As Albert Einstein said, "Insanity is doing the same thing over and over again and expecting different results." He also correctly pointed out that "the significant problems we face cannot be solved at the same level of thinking we were at when we created them". The bad eating habits many people have developed over the years have led many to become overweight. However, there is hope and new habits can be created and formed.

It all begins with us and the choices we make. We encourage you to make positive choices beginning today. You are the one who puts that food in your mouth. Others can recommend that you eat this or that, but ultimately, you are the one to decide what to eat. We have never heard anyone say that eating sugar is good for you. It may taste good in the moment, but that appears to be the only benefit it has. Are you going to allow the transient pleasure of eating sugary and fattening foods to deprive you of looking good and feeling great?

The beauty of the HCG program is that you do get to eat all of those sugary and fatty foods during your first two loading days without any quilt. Then for just a few weeks you limit yourself to the 500 calories/day. Since the HCG takes away most of your appetite and allows you to access your fat stores, this is not as hard as it sounds. After this phase you are able to eat a regular amount. We have found that after doing this program that we do not have the cravings we had before. Maybe this is a result of being completely off sugar for a few weeks or of having eaten so many of these fatty and sugary foods when we were loading and feeling very full as a result. Whatever the reason, we are grateful that this has been our experience.

Chapter 12

Conclusion

Bad habits are easier to abandon today than tomorrow.

—Yiddish saying

Dr. Simeons found that with the HCG in addition to the diet he recommended that just about every case of obesity and overweight can be handled successfully. However, he pointed out that it does require dedication and concentration and that it is better to follow this program as closely as you can. This is not a program that can be done half-heartedly without focusing on the details.

Obesity is a problem of epic proportions in the US. Being overweight can lead to many health challenges, as well as low self-esteem and emotional despair. Many people have tried many diets and programs to lose weight, as have we. Never have we seen a program that is so successful and results in such rapid weight loss when done correctly. It is for people who are ready and willing to follow this program as Dr. Simeons has recommended so that they may achieve their weight loss goals. The only thing you have to lose is unwanted fat and some bad habits. We hope you will begin today to look good and feel great.

We no longer believe that as you get older that you have to accept gaining weight. Nor do we believe that if you have not weighed a certain amount for more than two years that you can forget it. With Dr. Simeons' HCG program a person is able to reach their ideal weight, regardless of how long it has been (if ever) since they have weighed this. It is possible. We have done it as have hundreds of others we have known. At 50 we both happily weigh what we did in our twenties.

Dr. Simeons worked with thousands of patients and he has carefully and clearly determined how to do this program successfully. We are very grateful to him for his groundbreaking work. It is our great joy to be able to share this information with those who are seeking it and to make the homeopathic HCG drops available at our company website: www.ShiftingFrequencies.com

We would like you to have the body you have been wanting to have. It is our hope that you will set a course for an upward spiral in your own life so that your life can be all that you wish it to be. Whether you choose to do the HCG program or some other diet, we hope you will choose to do something to lose that extra weight. What do you have to lose except those unwanted pounds and inches?

The HCG program is one way to achieve your weight loss goals and to get in good shape. We have found it to be the best program for us and we have seen hundreds of others be successful with it as well. However, it is important to determine what is the best program for you. The main thing is that you do something. You can reach your ideal weight and avoid all of those weight-related illnesses that can lead some people to a downward spiral from which they are unable to recover. It is time to stop kicking yourself for the choices you have made in the past. Today is a new day and things can be different. We often remind ourselves that if we want things to be different, then we need to be different.

We wish you all the best on your journey and hope that you will make positive choices so that you can have the body you deserve to have and live the best life you are capable of living. Why wait another day to look and feel great?

Resources

Starting a new way of eating—new habits—can be a challenge. Many of the foods, supplements and sweeteners can be hard to find. The web site below provides some resources for where you can find HCG-related products.

ShiftingFrequencies.com

- HCG Homeopathic Drops
- Stevia Natural Sweetener Products
- DeLallo breadsticks
- Uncle Lee's Dieter's Tea (senna tea)

About the Authors

Felicia Weiss, Ph.D.

Felicia is a Licensed Clinical Psychologist, who focuses on wellness and personal growth. For almost twenty years, she has published the Holistic Networker magazine and produced the Wellness Expo® with her husband Tony. They also sell the HCG homeopathic drops and other related products online at ShiftingFrequencies.com.

Tony Cecala, Ph.D.

Tony is a business strategist specializing in technology solutions. While at Yale University, Tony earned two masters and a doctorate in Psychology. After graduation, he took a position at Texas Instruments in the *user-systems engineering* group. He designed both software and hardware systems for TI and presented research to upper management on trends in information technology.

He currently publishes the Holistic Networker magazine, produces the Wellness Expo®, and develops internet software solutions for business clients.